CARPAL TUNNEL SYNDROME:

How to Relieve and Prevent Wrist "Burnout"

by:

Rosemarie Atencio

CARPAL TUNNEL SYNDROME:

How to relieve & prevent wrist "BURNOUT"!

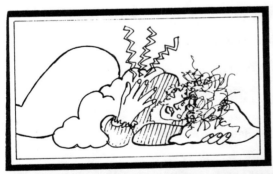
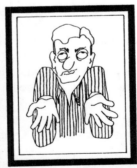

by Rosemarie Atencio

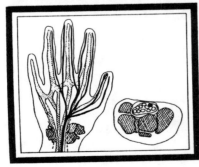
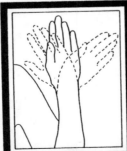
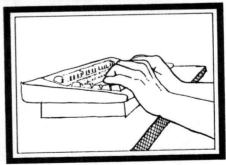

CARPAL TUNNEL SYNDROME:
How to Relieve and Prevent Wrist "Burnout" by Rosemarie Atencio

Published by: **HWD Publishing**
Post Office Box 220
Veneta, OR 97487

Publisher's Cataloging-in-Publication Data:
Atencio, Rosemarie
Carpal tunnel syndrome : how to relieve and prevent wrist "burnout"
/ by Rosemarie Atencio --- 1st ed
     p.   cm.
Includes index
1. Carpal tunnel syndrome. 2. Overuse injuries I. Title
RC422.C26
616.7'5, 616.8'7   93-79066

ISBN 0-9637360-1-9(pbk)

ACKNOWLEDGEMENTS

My deepest thanks to Dr. Sandra Ehsan, who in spite of a very serious illness, edited my material and always encouraged me. I also thank Dr. Sandra Simons who taught me about self-publishing. You showed much patience and interest.

A big thanks to Syd Skolsky who thought of me and called to say, "atta girl."

To my friends who read and edited text for me: Stan Hall, Phyllis Helland (thanks for the paste-up lesson), Linda Brown, and Dr. Gary Blair.

To all the people who entered the "Name the Book" contest. A special thanks to Enid Smith and Bob Shuken for the title to the last chapter.

To my models: Jan Cox, Mark Belden and Laurie Campbell - You looked mah-ve-lous. I also want to thank Jan and Elvis for many laughs.

Thanks to Dennis Hunt for marketing advice; to Steve Mayer for sharing the personnel department's viewpoint; to Nancy Cummings, Lynn Van Norman, LMT, and Mary Mitch, RN for the little boosts here and there.

My thanks to Linda Frazier for editing this book in record time. I also want to acknowledge Peter McCallum for the illustrations and cover.

ACKNOWLEDGEMENTS

To my friends and family who stayed in touch through this arduous process. Thanks to Jacquie, Jim and Mariella for never letting me get too intense. To all those who encouraged, helped and kept the faith - thank you.

TABLE OF CONTENTS

TABLE OF CONTENTS

TABLE OF CONTENTS

A WORD FROM ROSEMARIE

Through my private practice and consulting, I have heard many stories about loss of strength or feeling in the hands. I have talked to people who have had surgery and those who are trying to avoid it. The one overriding concern that I have heard time after time is: What can I do about it?

I have repeated this question to professionals in health and medicine. I have read quite a few books and magazine articles on the subject. From this research, I developed a workshop entitled, "It's All In the Wrists." Through these workshops, I reached some of the people who were concerned about relieving or preventing carpal tunnel syndrome. Yet, I knew there had to be a way to bring this information to more people.

That is how this book came to be. I couldn't find a book for the consumer on carpal tunnel syndrome at the public library nor at the university library. What I did find on the topic was either a medical book, an ergonomic book, or a book directed only to professionals.

This book is neither a medical book nor an ergonomic book. I have tried to avoid the use of medical or anatomical terms. Where I could not avoid the use of a medical term, I have defined it in either the text or the glossary.

A WORD FROM ROSEMARIE

Professionals may take exception to some points, and I welcome their comments. However, this book is intended primarily for the layperson.

The book's margins are wide so that, if it is your personal book or you are using it in conjunction with my workshop, you will have room to make notes. Also, I strived to make the book "user friendly." At different stages in the development of this book, I would ask clients and friends for their opinion. I even conducted an informal survey to choose the cover. I did not want this book to be a chore to read. Please write to the publisher's address and let me know your thoughts, ideas and outcomes after reading this book.

I did limit this book to carpal tunnel syndrome, and did not go into any depth about the problems that may arise from the shoulder or neck. My decision not to expand the book was twofold: (1) Sheer size may have discouraged people from reading it, and (2) People with shoulder or neck problems do not necessarily have wrist/hand complaints, and people with true CTS do not need to read about neck and shoulders.

Above all, my objective in writing this book was to give readers the tools to take care of themselves.

Wishing you the joy of good health,

Rosemarie Atencio, HHP,LMT
August 1993

REASONS

and

CAUSES

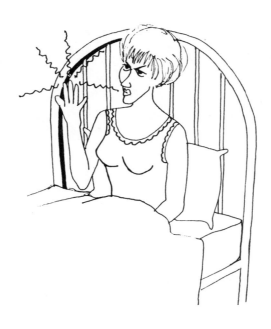

Chapter 1

THE MAGIC TOUCH

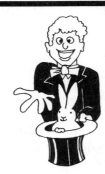 Once upon a time, there was a magician who was famous for his great acts of magic. He was asked by his apprentice how he was able to be so proficient - so deft - at his hand movement. The magician shrugged his shoulders and said: "It's simple. It's all in the wrists."

The idea of the wrists being important in the control of movement is not so farfetched. The wrists, forearms, hands and fingers provide us with the movement that enables us to do everything from fixing the plumbing to playing the piano to constructing magnificent cathedrals. This great range of movement and dexterity has allowed us to create the world that we enjoy today.

 So, what would life be like without the movement and dexterity that we depend upon?

Imagine a life in which your fingers go numb at night and you wake up with tingling in your hands. Imagine being unable to tie your shoes or even to grasp the shoelace between your fingers and thumb. Imagine not being able to distinguish hot from cold in your fingers. Imagine feeling pain in your hands whenever you try to move or manipulate something.

Section I: REASONS AND CAUSES

Some of those symptoms could be a description of arthritis, or diabetes or other ailments listed in Chapter 2. More often, it is a description of an advanced case of carpal tunnel syndrome.

It is not a pretty picture, but neither is it a hopeless one. There is much that you can do to prevent loss of the integrity of your wrists and hands. This book is about prevention and relief. You will learn, as you read this, what you can do to maintain the natural integrity of your wrists, hands and fingers.

Companies hire me to provide workshops for their staff and to observe and consult with the staff on the prevention of injuries including carpal tunnel syndrome. Why are companies so interested in prevention? The reason is that companies have found that prevention reduces their medical costs and absenteeism while increasing morale and productivity. I have had the benefit of feedback from many people.

If companies realize it is cheaper to buy prevention through education than to pay for injuries, it makes dollars and sense *for you, too.*

Carpal tunnel syndrome does not play favorites or occur in only one setting, one job, or one hobby. I hear from people in all walks of life: hairdressers who no

Chapter 1: THE MAGIC TOUCH

longer have the strength in their hands to cut hair; assembly workers who have had to change jobs, and musicians who don't know how they can continue to play. I have spoken to homemakers, writers and carpenters. The list is long. Some have had surgery, others are denying or avoiding their symptoms for as long as possible and others simply do not understand what they are experiencing.

 Take heart. You can be effective. If you have the symptoms or want to prevent them, there are many things that you can do. Don't give up without trying. There are choices that won't involve a dramatic change in your lifestyle. You do need to commit to taking care of yourself.

After you finish reading this book, you will know how to pay attention to your body movements and placement. You will know how to keep up with the prevention techniques that work for you. The information that I am giving you is the same information that I provide to employees at workshops and in my consulting practice. So let's get started on your journey of self-care. Read and do the exercises provided. You'll have fun while you learn.

Chapter 2

WHY ME?

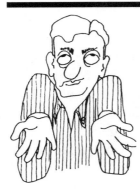

When unfortunate things happen to us, we often wonder why. This book would not be complete without a chapter on the reasons for carpal tunnel syndrome. Perhaps the best way to explain the reasons for carpal tunnel syndrome is to divide them into groups.

For the purposes of this book, let's look at the groups in terms of the following divisions:

(1) **<u>Congenital reasons</u>**
These are the physically unique situations that exist at birth. In this category, are people who are born with small carpal tunnels as well as those whose muscles or nerves may have formed a little differently. People who have these naturally occuring conditions need to pay particular attention to posture, movement, muscle exhaustion, and a tendency to overcompensate.

(2) **<u>Self-limiting reasons</u>**
These are the conditions such as pregnancy or in-jury in which time will be the limiting factor of a

carpal tunnel problem. Since time and nature will take care of the problem, the best advice is to be patient and try not to "plow through."

3 **Systemic reasons**
These are illnesses which affect the body generally. This group includes diseases such as: rheumatoid arthritis, diabetes, tumors, gout, edema, and hypothyroidism, which affects joints, circulation and nerves. Almost everyone in this category is under medical care. In addition to medical treatment, a good diet and sufficient rest, as described further in this book, can help to relieve symptoms.

4 **Non-medical reasons**
This is the category for incorrect posture, poorly designed work stations and/or tools, low room temperatures, high repetition, high vibration, excessive use of force, or insufficient rest. This group can benefit most by becoming aware of their movements, taking mini-vacations (as described later in this book), and practicing prevention.

(There have been some studies that also point to women

Section I: REASONS AND CAUSES

---

as being more susceptible. Since women are employed more often for highly repetitive tasks such as data entry, small parts assembling and cold packing work, they are generally at somewhat greater risk.)

As you read through the categories one through four, did you find at least one area that described your situation? Know this:

No matter what category you are in, there will be suggestions in this book that can help you.

Chapter 3

IN THE GOOD OLE DAYS

Have you ever wondered how in days gone by, someone could bang on one of those plain, old, non-electric type-writers all day and not wind up with carpal tunnel problems? After all, it took lots of finger force on those manual typewriters. And like today, people would sit and work at their stations all day long. Yet, there weren't near the number of carpal tunnel syndrome cases then as there are now. Why is that?

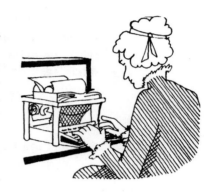

Several reasons can be given. First, there was a variety of movements. Second, the movements required the fingers and wrists to be strong. Third, the action could only continue until the bottom of a single page.

Let's look at what would happen today if every time you wanted to print a page, you had to feed it into the printer. First of all, you would have to stop entering data. Then, you would have to pick up a piece of paper and place it in the printer and push the button to feed the paper into the printer. Next, you would have to go through a sequence of button pushing on the keyboard to begin printing. As soon as that page was printed, you would have to put in another page and then another and so on.

Section I: REASONS AND CAUSES

What would be happening is that there would be enough variety of movement to keep the wrist, forearms, hands and fingers from remaining too long at the same task in the same stressful position. Not only would you have avoided long hours of repetition, but your wrist, hands and fingers would have enjoyed a sort of rest or respite (mini-vacation) from the process of punching keys continuously.

 MINI-VACATIONS:
A small rest, an exercise, or another task that breaks up the cycles of repetitive work.

When I mention sufficient rest, I don't necessarily mean taking your breaks (which matter, too). I am talking about varying your tasks and the small stops that you build into your work pattern to give the body a variety of movement.

When jobs became more repetitive and competitive, we did not understand the impact on the body. We need to retreat from the notion that the body can sit or stand or do the same motion for long periods of time.

Chapter 3: IN THE GOOD OLE DAYS

You were meant to move. A full 40 percent of you is muscle, and the only function of muscle is movement. The hands alone can make 56 distinctively different movements. Using only a small portion of the muscles over and over again tends to fatigue the muscle. When a muscle fatigues, it needs time to regenerate itself. This process of regeneration is what our muscles are doing when we rest.

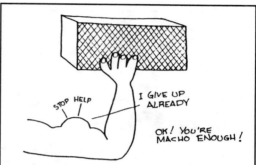

Using only a small portion of the muscle over and over again tends to fatigue the muscle.

Let's look at the group of people that need quick regeneration of the muscles the most - the athletes. Gone are the days when athletes exercised in the same way day after day. Today, the typical athlete's schedule looks like this: Monday, Wednesday and Friday may involve weight training for resistance and to build bulk. The other days are devoted to aerobics for greater cardiovascular efficiency.

Most professional athletes also have alternate ways of exercising built into their routine so that if their muscles begin to fatigue, they can do something else. For

Section I: Reasons and Causes

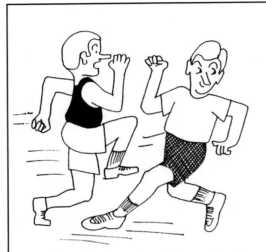

If athletes begin to tire while running forward, they use other muscles by turning around and running backwards.

example, on a cardio-vascular workout day, the athlete may alternate between running and walking or may turn around and run backwards.

What have trainers learned about optimizing the training of an elite athlete that could apply to all of us? What these trainers have learned is that when you use a muscle, it tears down muscle tissue. I know that "tears down" sounds dramatic, but that is what actually happens to the muscle. When the muscle isn't given time to build back up, it becomes inflamed from overuse. *Overuse leads to injury.*

When the muscles and tendons that pass through the carpal tunnel become inflamed from overuse or misuse, they pinch the nerve. It's kind of like the cowboy saying, "There ain't enough room in this town for the both of us."

Muscles need time to rest and regenerate. Not only do you need to get sufficient sleep, but you also need to build enough variety into your routine to keep the muscles from becoming overly fatigued.

Muscle Use + Insufficient Rest = Inflammation and Injury

Try not to get yourself so deeply involved in your home chores, job, or hobbies that you exceed the stamina of your muscles. Take time every half hour to get up and do something else. Stretch, get a drink of water, take a deep breath. Actually, those mini-vacations can also clear your mind so that you can return to what you were doing and feel even more alert.

Chapter 4

I AIN'T GOT NO BODY

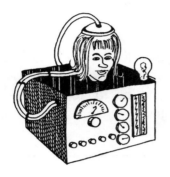

When we suffer an injury or we feel ill, we think that somehow our body has betrayed us. The opposite is usually true. It is our belief in the body as a servant of the mind that keeps us from paying attention to early signs of illness or pain.

In my workshops, I tell participants that our attitude about our bodies reminds me of a certain science fiction movie. Perhaps you've seen it. In the movie, a woman is in a horrible accident and all that remains of her is her head. Her head is hooked up to all sorts of bells and whistles and she can see, talk, and hear just fine. She doesn't seem to need a body at all.

Most of us are living as talking heads. In other words, we have become divorced from our bodies. We do not want to deal with its nagging and demanding ways. We want our body to conform to what we tell it to do when we want it done - and no back talk. It seems that we need to experience a great deal of discomfort or pain before we become sufficiently alarmed to do something about our physical selves.

Chapter 4: I AIN'T GOT NO BODY

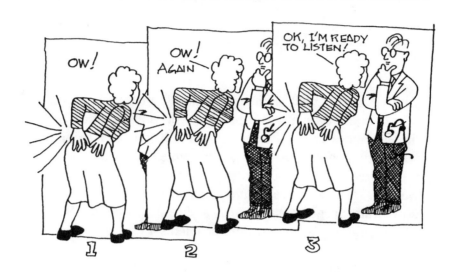

For example, a client told me that she has suffered a stabbing muscle spasm in her back. It was so painful that she could barely stand upright. She went to the doctor. The doctor told her what she needed to do to prevent the problem from occurring again. He also told her that he knew once she was out of pain, she would not follow through. He said that was OK with him because he was prepared to tell her two more times. That is, when she came back the next time with muscle spasms, and when she came back the third time for the same reason. He knew that the third time she suffered the pain would be the first time she would listen. By the third time, the possibility of another occurrence would

Section I: REASONS AND CAUSES

be so intimidating that she would take action to prevent it from happening a fourth time.

Don't worry about someone thinking that you are a hypochondriac or a wimp because you pay attention to those twinges and sensations of pain. **It is better to act when the problem is new.** Acting when the problem is acute (usually considered to persist less than two weeks), gives you a better chance of stopping the downward progression towards a chronic problem. (See facing page regarding chronic problems.)

You may feel that you haven't any problems now. Good for you. Keep in mind that if you are in a high risk job or have a predisposing condition (such as I described in Chapter 2), prevention is the kindest act you can do for yourself. Never take good health for granted. It is a gift that comes to us with responsibility. I have a workshop titled: "If I Wear Out My Body, Where Will I Live?" Think about it: How *long* do you plan to live in your body? And how *well* do you plan to live in your body?

Many physical movements are done without considering what happens to our body over time. I say "over time" because when we are very young, we bounce

Chapter 4: I AIN'T GOT NO BODY

What Happens to Us When We Have a "Chronic Problem?"

To answer that, let's look at the way a problem grows if we ignore it:

(a) The longer that healthy parts have to compensate for the part that has discomfort or pain, the more involvement the healthy muscles, tendons and bones will have in the problem.

(b) The longer the problem is allowed to continue, the greater the likelihood that the treatment will be the most dramatic that medicine has to offer.

(c) The longer that discomfort or pain is endured, the less patience there will be in searching out the least invasive option.

(d) The longer that the problem continues, the longer it will take to heal once treatment begins

(e) The longer it takes to heal, the more the feelings of uselessness and depression persist.

(You could probably add a few statements of your own on the results of waiting too long.)

Section I: REASONS AND CAUSES

back rapidly. In time, the accumulation of repetitive motions and poor posture take their toll. This is true for most of the problems of the wrist. *Symptoms occur because we have been doing something for so long or so repeatedly that our hands, wrists and fingers can no longer tolerate the action.*

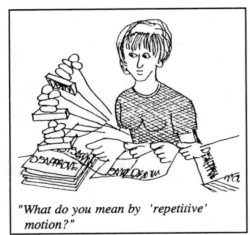

"What do you mean by 'repetitive' motion?"

These type of injuries are known in the health profession as "repetitive motion injuries" or "cumulative trauma disorders" or a host of other names. What these expressions mean is that for one reason or another, you have been doing the wrong movement repeatedly - or doing the right movement but without sufficient rest.

The wrong movement can be caused by your posture or your work station. On the other hand (no pun intended), your posture and work station may be fine. However, you work too long without rest and go beyond the stamina of your muscles.

Chapter 4: I AIN'T GOT NO BODY

The reason for providing you with this information is to help you build body awareness. You need to know what your body is doing in response to your request that a movement be one way or the other. Notice your body. Since this book is about the carpal tunnel, let's begin with your wrists, hands and fingers.

SECTION II

HEALTH

and

MEDICINE

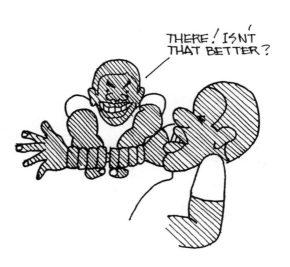

THERE! ISN'T THAT BETTER?

Chapter 5

Who's on First? What's a Carpal? and Other Little Known Facts

In baseball, before we can get to first base, we had to complete a great deal of preparation and practice. We had to learn to use a bat properly. We had to learn to hit a ball with the bat. We had to learn the rules of the game. The same holds true for learning how to prevent problems with our wrists. If we are going to learn how to take care of ourselves, we have to learn something about the way we tick.

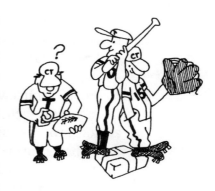

We'll start with the most inner layer, the bones, and work our way out. There are eight small bones in the wrist which are called the "carpals." They are shaped roughly like small squares with rounded edges which fit together like a stone arch. The mortar is provided by cartilage between the bones. The design is ingenious.

The carpals provide rigidity while allowing for a greater degree of flexibility than a solid bone or a single joint can provide. This allows us to move

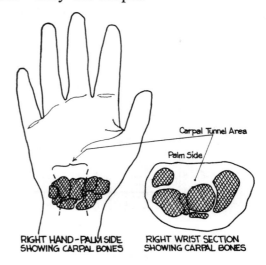

Carpal Tunnel Area

Palm Side

RIGHT HAND - PALM SIDE
SHOWING CARPAL BONES

RIGHT WRIST SECTION
SHOWING CARPAL BONES

Section II: HEALTH AND MEDICINE

our wrists up and down and, to a lesser degree, from side to side. Go ahead and move your wrists up and down and then side to side so that you can feel the full range of movement.

Bones are the framework that holds us up but bones cannot move on their own. Remember the skeleton in the anatomy or biology class at school? Do you remember what happened when you took the skeleton off the hanger? You're right. It collapsed. That's because bones provide rigidity but not movement or tension. What provides the body with movement and tension are the muscles and tendons.

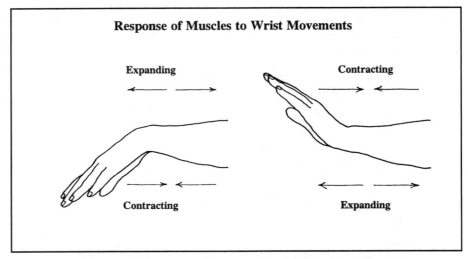

Muscle expands and contracts to provide movement and tension

Chapter 5: WHO'S ON FIRST?...

Muscles contract and expand to provide movement in the hands and fingers. Most of these muscles are located in your forearm. Place your hand on the forearm of your other hand about an inch below your elbow joint and make a fist. Then roll that fist in towards your wrist as far as you can. Now, roll your fist as far as possible in the other direction. Can you feel the movement in your forearm? The muscles are like a puppeteer's hands, the tendons are like his strings, and the bones are like his puppet. As the puppeteer (muscle) tugs on the string (tendon), the puppet (bone) moves.

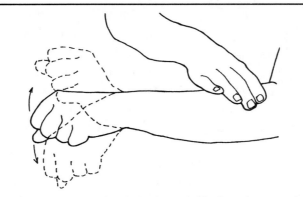

1. *Place one hand on the opposite forearm an inch below your elbow and make a fist.*
2. *Roll your fist in towards your wrist.*
3. *Now, roll your fist in the other direction as far as you can.*

Section II: HEALTH AND MEDICINE

Feel your wrist. The bones can be felt right under the skin. How do those tendons coming from the muscles in the forearm get to their destination at the fingers and thumb when the wrist is such a narrow part of the body?

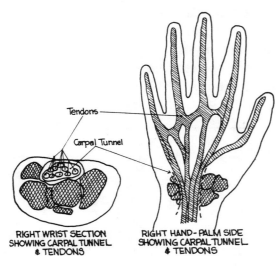

Tendons

Carpal Tunnel

RIGHT WRIST SECTION
SHOWING CARPAL TUNNEL
& TENDONS

RIGHT HAND- PALM SIDE
SHOWING CARPAL TUNNEL
& TENDONS

The answer is that the carpals fit together to make an upside down arch on the palm side of your wrist. You can feel it right at the base of the palm. Push the area at the bottom of the palm where the palm meets the wrist. That space is where nine of the tendons (puppet strings) pass through on their way to generate movement of the fingers and thumb.

Since there is not a lot of room in the hand, fingers and wrist, the tendons need a way of staying separated as they pass through the same small opening. They also need a way of staying lubricated for movement. This is

Chapter 5: WHO'S ON FIRST?...

accomplished by a sheath around each tendon called the "synovial sheath."

There is one more important player that you need to know about: the nerves. There are three main nerves that exit the spinal column at the neck, pass under the collarbone and shoulder, run down the arm and into the hand. One of them, called the "median" or middle nerve, also passes through the same arch as the nine tendons mentioned in the previous paragraph.

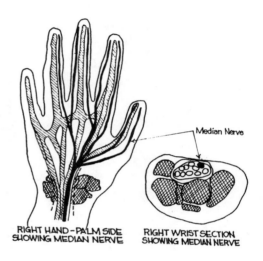

RIGHT HAND - PALM SIDE
SHOWING MEDIAN NERVE

RIGHT WRIST SECTION
SHOWING MEDIAN NERVE

So far, I have been telling you about an arch, so where is the tunnel? In order to provide stability and give more strength to the wrist, there is a ligament of tough fibrous tissue that wraps around the wrist. That is how the arch becomes a tunnel. With the hand turned palm side up, the carpals (bones) form the floor and part of the sides of the tunnel while the ligament forms the rest of the sides and ceiling of the tunnel.

The picture is now complete: the tunnel is made up of the arched carpal bones and the carpal ligament. Running through the tunnel are the sheathed tendons and the median nerve.

Congratulations! You have just completed your anatomy lesson.

Review of the Carpal Tunnel

Try your "hand" at identifying the names of the anatomy parts that make up the tunnel...(answers are at the bottom of the page)

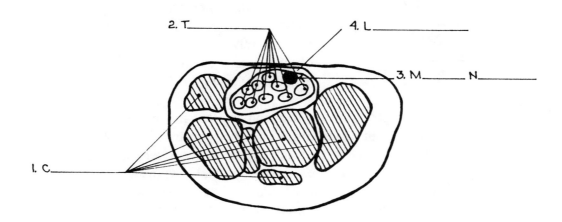

2. T_____   4. L_____

3. M_____   N_____

I. C_____

1. Carpals
2. Tendons
3. Median Nerve
4. Ligament

Chapter 6

I GOTTA RIGHT TO SING THE BLUES

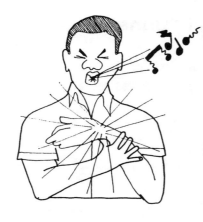

We've looked at the word "carpal" and the word "tunnel," now let's look at the word "syndrome." A syndrome is based on signs and symptoms that seem to add up to a certain problem in our body. In other words, when a doctor notices something wrong, it is called a "sign." When you describe your observations to the doctor, it is called a "symptom."

We can put it all together and say that in simple terms, carpal tunnel syndrome means that you have something going on in the wrist tunnel. That is not a very definite diagnosis. You see, carpal tunnel syndrome like "whiplash," "frozen shoulder," "water on the knees" and a few other common names does not define the source of the problem. That's a lot tougher to figure out. Let's look at the problems with proper diagnosis.

Suppose you are waking up at night with numbness or tingling running down to your little finger. Do you have carpal tunnel syndrome? The answer is "no." That isn't to say that you do not have a problem, it just

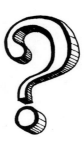

means that the nerve being affected is not passing through the carpal tunnel. You see, there are other nerves and tendons that work the hand and fingers but do not go through the tunnel. Therefore, part of the diagnosis is determining which nerve is being affected. Sometimes this can be ascertained by knowing which fingers are experiencing the discomfort

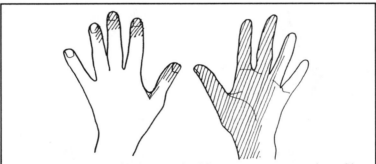

Pain or discomfort often occurs in this area or some portion of it when the median nerve is involved.

Along with finding which nerve branch is involved, the question is why the nerve is sending tingling or numbness signals into the hand. This is made more difficult because of the route that the nerves travel to get to the hand and fingers. As I stated in an earlier chapter, the nerves exit the spine from the neck, pass under the collarbone as well as the shoulder and run

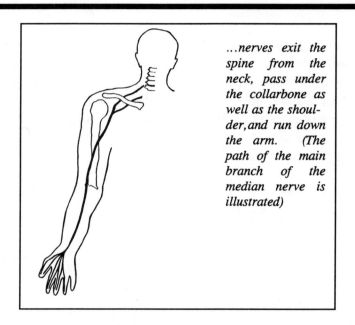

...nerves exit the spine from the neck, pass under the collarbone as well as the shoulder, and run down the arm. (The path of the main branch of the median nerve is illustrated)

down the arm to the hand The possibility of an impingement ("pinched nerve") exists anywhere along the nerve pathways. For example, when muscles and tendons expand through inflammation, they can press on nerves; resting your elbow on a hard surface can pinch off a nerve. So can resting your wrist on a sharp edge. *This problem of the pain being noticed in one place and the cause being somewhere else is known as "referred pain."* Referred pain can make proper diagnosis very difficult. (The problems of the head, neck, upper back and shoulders are so extensive that they will be the subjects of subsequent books).

Chapter 6: I GOTTA RIGHT...

When numbness or tingling is reported in the hands or fingers, carpal tunnel syndrome is often given as the diagnosis. Don't be too hasty in accepting that diagnosis. The problem might be thoracic outlet syndrome, pronator teres syndrome, or flexor tenosynovitis - to name a few other possibilities. Accurate diagnosis is tricky. You need to be aware that you could spend a lot of discouraging time and money on a misdiagnosis.

What are you to do? State-of-the-art clinical assessment is changing so rapidly that mention of any particular method would make this book outdated before it was published. My advice is to be a thoughtful consumer. You don't take your car to a quick lube place to rebuild your car's transmission. You go to a specialist. Why would you do anything less for your body?

Find the doctor who specializes in carpal tunnel syndrome and related problems. Ask the same questions that you ask for the care and repair of your car. Start

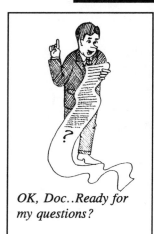

OK, Doc..Ready for my questions?

by putting your symptoms and questions on paper BEFORE your appointment. At the interview, listen, listen and listen. If you feel that the doctor has the experience and compassion you want, then you are probably with the right professional. Above all, remember that you are the consumer.

Chapter 6: I GOTTA RIGHT...

IF YOU NEED TO SEE A PROFESSIONAL:

1 On a piece of paper, write a list of your symptoms. Here are questions for you to consider:

- ❑   What are the sensations?
- ❑   Where are these sensations?
- ❑   What time of day do the symptoms occur?
- ❑   What are you doing at the time that you have symptoms (asleep, specific movement at work..) ?
- ❑   What makes you feel better?
- ❑   What makes you feel worse?
- ❑   What treatment(s) (drugs, splinting, etc) have you tried that did not work?
- ❑   How long did you stay on the treatment?
- ❑   How long have you had the problem?

(In addition to the specific symptoms, you need to be prepared to briefly describe any traumas or accidents that you may have had to the neck, shoulders, arms and hands.)

Section II: HEALTH AND MEDICINE

2 On the same piece of paper, write down the information about your lifestyle and job.

- ❑ What physical actions are required on your job?
- ❑ What are your hobbies?
- ❑ What kind of physical activities do you do regularly?
- ❑ Do you participate in any sports?
- ❑ Do you sleep well?
- ❑ Do you eat well?
- ❑ Do you take any drugs or supplements?

3 Finally, list the questions that you have about the professional people and the course of treatment that recommended. (Be bold! You are the consumer.)

- ❑ How long have they worked with cumulative trauma or repetitive motion disorders?
- ❑ What is the course of treatment that they recommend for such disorders?
- ❑ How do they feel about second opinions?

Chapter 6: I GOTTA RIGHT...

❑   How do they feel about cooperating with other professionals (physical therapists, acupuncturists, osteopaths, for example)?

❑   What results would they consider satisfactory?

❑   How long would they continue a specific course of treatment?

❑   If surgery is required, what arrangements do they have for after-care?

Use these questions as a guide. Make up some of your own. Think seriously about the concerns that you have about your job, the use of your hands and fingers, and the time and effort it will take to get better. *Be sure to write down ALL your questions.* That way, when you have those precious few minutes to talk to the professional, you will be able to quickly get to the point of your visit. It is better to ask questions at the visit rather than to call back and wait for the nurse/doctor/ therapist to get back to you.

Chapter 7

DOOR NUMBER ONE, DOOR NUMBER TWO OR DOOR NUMBER THREE?

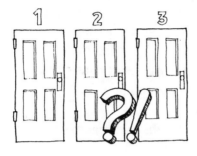

Even though the goal of this book is relief and prevention, it is important to know what medical or health treatments are available. With this information, you can take an active part in your health care.

Let's say that the diagnosis is carpal tunnel syndrome. What can be done medically? At the extreme end, when all else has failed to bring relief, you can have surgery. High numbers of people do get relief with surgical intervention, but *have a return of symptoms within 3 to 5 years*. It seems that even though the surgery has made the tunnel larger, the tendons can swell and fill the enlarged tunnel and once again press on the nerve. Another problem that can occur after surgery is a loss of power in the grip of the hand, thumb, or finger. Sometimes, there is persistent pain, or a loss in finger sensation, or an increased sensitivity in the palms after surgery.

For many people, returning to the job that they previously had is impossible. If they are able to do the same job at all, it is only for part of the day. In order to

---

function at work, they need to be given other tasks or possibly another job. (The question is, if they had changed jobs or tasks in the first place, could they have avoided surgery?)

Leaving the more radical approach of surgery, but staying in the medical mode, the doctor may offer steroid injections or an anti-inflammatory drug. These treatments may help in the short run, but cannot be used indefinitely. You need to identify the techniques that you can use to prevent the problem from occurring again or to keep the problem from getting worse.

Sometimes the doctor or employer will want you to use a splint. Splints come in many sizes and shapes. Some are movement or job specific. Splinting may be necessary when the area needs to be immobilized. A splint, like medication, may be helpful but should not be relied upon indefinitely. Muscles, tendons and joints need to work to become

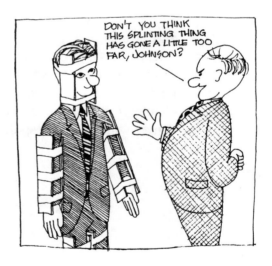

strong. The longer that the splint is used, the weaker and more accident prone the body becomes.

Another possibility after diagnosis is a trip to a therapist. Depending on the diagnosis, the therapist could be a physical therapist or a massage therapist. Again, referring back to the example of your car, make sure that the therapist has the experience you need. Part of your therapy needs to include a plan to teach you preventive measures. It is not enough to have a therapy session and then set up another appointment. You need to be given information about changes in your lifestyle, posture and job to help you learn to take care of yourself.

Since surgery provides mixed results and drugs and splints have limited effectiveness, you need to practice awareness and prevention. It is your best bet. As I said in an earlier chapter, good health is a gift that comes with certain responsibilities.

RELIEF

and

PREVENTION

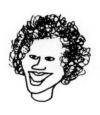

Chapter 8

I AM *NOT* IN A BAD MOOD

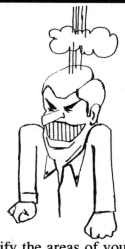

No discussion in prevention would cover the bases without taking up the subject of stress. I could write indefinitely about the role of high levels of stress as a causal factor in any illness. High levels of stress are those heavy-duty-no-time-for-me relentless stresses that take a great toll on us.

 Whether or not you can identify the areas of your life that are the source of your stress, there is one thing I can tell you for certain: **eventually the results of continuous stress will show up in your body.** So, while you are sorting out other phases of your life, you need to be taking care of your physical self.

To understand the involvement of the physical self in stress, let's spend a minute in "the loop:" you have an end-of-the-month deadline - that's a stressor. Your body wants to leave the computer for awhile but you say "No. There's no time now, " - there is another stressor. You are getting achy and then someone says something that irritates and bingo! - another stressor. You don't have to be Einstein to realize what happens next. Yes, you meet the deadline but right after that, you come down with (your choice of illness in this space.) You are home in bed and you are even further behind in your work. (Well, it was the only way your body/mind could get you to stop.) You try to get back to work as soon as you can to start the whole cycle all over again. You are in the loop of head stress, followed by body stress, followed by more head stress, followed by more body stress.

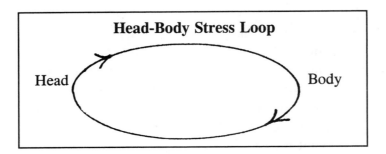

Head-Body Stress Loop

Head   Body

Sometimes the stress loop starts at a physical level. You might be working hard and getting things done. You are feeling good about your accomplishments. Your body has been resistant to the pace, but you are on a mental high. You do not want to stop. However, you are waking up at night because you are having tingling or numbness in your fingers or hands. You are concerned about what is happening to you physically

Chapter 8: I AM *NOT IN* A BAD MOOD

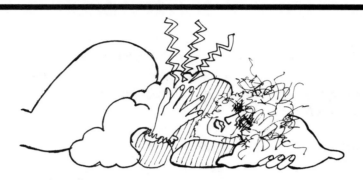

and you are tired because you didn't sleep well. You know that you are beginning to experience a physical component of stress and you don't like it. You do not want to have to deal with it. Now, with the lack of sleep and the worry about your health, you go out to face the day. It does not take much for some yahoo to upset you. This time, the physical stress had led to a mental/emotional stress.

How well can you live with underlying worry and doubts about your health? Do you want to step out of "the loop?"

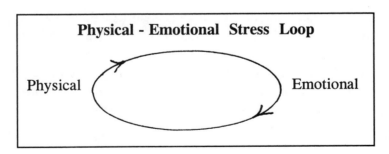

Section III: RELIEF AND PREVENTION

Begin now by taking a quick physical inventory. Are you overriding any places in your body that have pain or discomfort? Are you dismissing a small physical discomfort?

Whatever you do, don't ignore yourself. Forget the concern that someone might think you are a hypochondriac. (Which reminds me of the tombstone that read, "See, I told you I was sick.") *Small, nagging pains matter.* Usually pain is a signal that you need to stop whatever it is that is causing aggravation. Maybe you need to learn to do it differently.

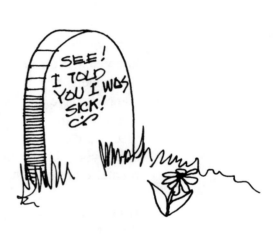

I have heard all the arguments against taking care of oneself - including the argument that the time to learn will slow you down. Yes, while you are learning new ways, you will slow down a little, but you will learn what is a good pace for you. You will learn preventive measures to keep yourself out of the stress loop.

Chapter 8: I AM *NOT* IN A BAD MOOD

No one knows your body better than you do. Decide now to learn to treat yourself well. Learn the subtle things your body likes. Generally, the demands aren't great - wholesome food, some activity everyday, sufficient rest and lots of laughter.

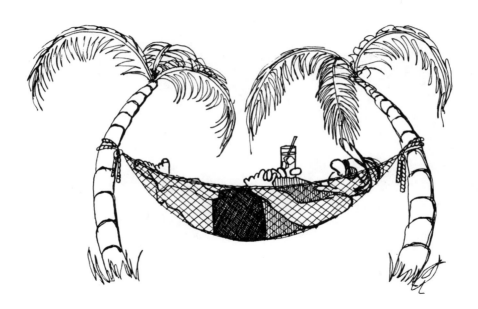

Chapter 8: I AM *NOT* IN A BAD MOOD

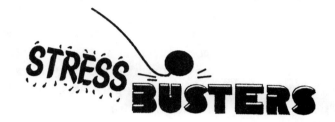

O Try not to set unrealistic, perfectionistic standards for yourself.

O Let off steam with physical activity.

O Before eating or drinking anything, ask yourself if you are really hungry or thirsty. If not, go for a walk instead.

O Do some belly breathing everytime you feel stressed. Expand your belly when you inhale and let the breath out very slowly. Do this 5-10 times.

O Get out of the stress loop by doing something nice for someone else - without expectations of getting anything other than a good feeling.

O LAUGH ALOT!

Chapter 9

STAYING IN NEUTRAL

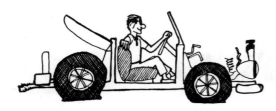

With the body, there is a "best" position. That is to say there is a position which the body likes best because it generates the least amount of strain on the muscles, tendons and joints.

Using the wrist as an example, if you were to extend your forearm and wrist so that there is a straight line down the arm, the hand and the fingers, this would be considered the neutral position. In other words, this position puts the least amount of work on the wrist joint.

As you move the wrist from side to side or up and down, you increase the angle of the joint. Try this: first, bend your wrist down towards your arm; then extend your hand upwards. Can you feel the strain at the limitation of the wrist joint ?

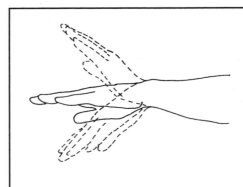

From the neutral position, move your hand up. (This is called "extension.") and then move your hand down. (This is called "flexion.") Note the strain at the limitation of the wrist joint.

Chapter 9: STAYING IN NEUTRAL...

Let's try the other two moves of the wrist: move your hand so that it angles towards the thumb. Now move it in the opposite direction towards your little finger. Did you notice the limit of the range of motion and some pulling on the muscles? The further away from neutral or the more frequently we deviate from neutral, the more effort we put on the joint and muscles.

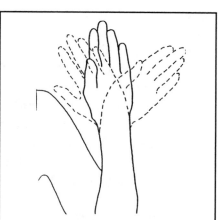

Angle your hand towards your thumb ("radial" side). Move in the opposite direction towards your little finger ("ulnar" side). Notice the limitation.

I have a friend who was having trouble with her wrist and she could not understand why. As it happens, she carried a fairly heavy briefcase. Every time she lifted the briefcase to place it on her desk or some other surface, she gave the movement a little "English"- which is to say that she was giving a flick of her wrist at the end of the movement. The weight of the briefcase and movement from neutral that the extra flick provided were putting additional stress on her wrist joint, muscles and tendons.

Section III: RELIEF AND PREVENTION

The computer keyboard is a good example of how we deviate from the neutral wrist position. If you tend to hit the return or the shift or any of the other keys that are not directly in front of you by a flick of the wrist, the high repetition of this movement can bring discomfort at the end of a day. Even though I have used the computer keyboard to illustrate the point, there are other jobs where this tendency occurs. I have observed supermarket checkers putting a little flick at the end of their movements. Almost any wrist movement can involve a little "English." *Check out your own motions and see if that extra flick of the wrist is at the base of your wrist problem.*

This is a very important point: you don't have to make sweeping movements to cause stress on the wrist. A small but highly repetitive incorrect movement can aggravate the joint and all of the muscles that go into making the move. The muscle and tendon can become inflamed and impinge on the nerve.

In addition to repetition that stresses the wrists and muscles from side to side, I have observed that many workers work with their wrists bent upward or

Chapter 9: STAYING IN NEUTRAL

downward. Repetitive downward motion is often noticeable with certain tasks such as the hand packing of boxes. The upward bending motion is frequently found when workers rest their wrist on a surface thereby forcing their hand upwards.

NOTE: In the upward bent position, the hand should not be more than 15 degrees higher than the wrist.

I like the image that was expressed to me by someone who had taken a martial art class. The teacher said that when you bend the wrist, energy gets stuck and cannot carry down the arm and off the hand and fingers. That description of "stuck" energy could also apply to the inflamed muscles and tendons that impinge on the nerve.

Observe your movements while doing a repetitive task. Notice the position of your hands and wrists. Are your wrists straight in all directions? Or are you resting your wrists on the desk, tabletop, or other surface thereby forcing your wrists to bend? If you are doing assembly work or using tools, what repetitive motions move the wrist away from neutral and what can you do to correct the movement? Can you place your tools or equipment in a way that works better for you?

Page 67

Section III: RELIEF AND PREVENTION

When I was learning massage, I thought that I would be unable to do massages all day because my arms and thumbs ached so much by the end of a day. Once I identified the movement which was causing the problem and corrected my motions, I stopped having any achiness or soreness. I was able to work on six to eight clients in a day in comfort.

Before we leave the subject of wrist deviation, I have a couple of questions for you: (1) Do you sleep with your wrist curled under? (2) Do you like to sleep with your arm tucked under the pillow and your head resting on it? There are doctors who believe that these sleeping postures tend to aggravate the CTS condition.

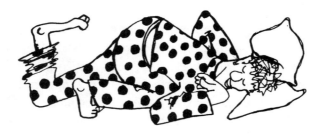

You probably don't want to wake up during the night in order to note your sleep position, right? Then the answer for you may be to wear a splint at night.

Since we all like to sleep comfortably and without restrictions, you will want to find a splint made out of a light weight material. You do not need a heavy duty one that is made for work. The splint should have a small hard piece at the junction of the wrist and the palm of sufficient stiffness to keep the wrist straight. There are so many types of splints that you will not find it difficult to locate one that allows you to sleep comfortably and at the same time prevents those wrist curling movements.

Section III: RELIEF AND PREVENTION

WHAT'S WRONG WITH THESE PICTURES?

Now that you have completed the chapter, see if you can identify the incorrect movement(s) in these pictures: (Answers are on the next page.)

Terms: *radial:* towards thumb, *ulnar:* towards little finger, *extension:* hand bending up, *flexion:* hand bending down

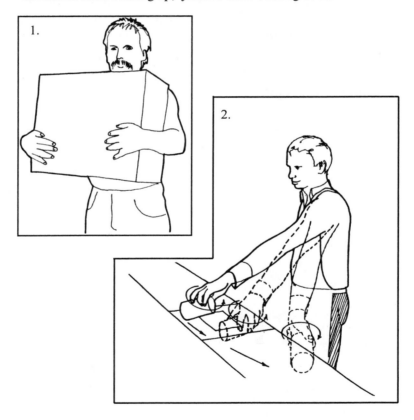

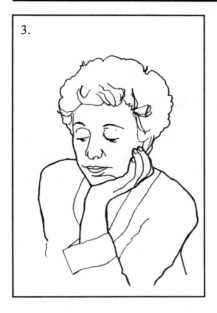

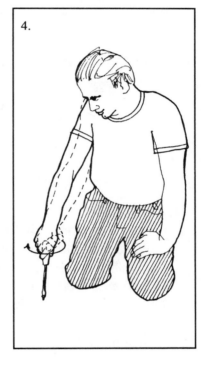

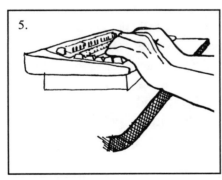

1. Flexion (compression at wrist)
2. Ulnar deviation
3. Extension (compression at elbow)
4. Ulnar deviation
5. Extension, radial deviation (compression at wrists.)

Chapter 10

A BETTER POSITION

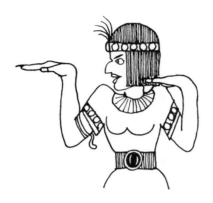

Once you have observed your wrist movement, the next thing you want to do is look at your overall shoulder, arm and wrist posture. The placement of your shoulders and arms are also major players in your hand and wrist comfort.

The most comfortable position for the arms and shoulders is as follows:

1. Shoulders should be relaxed. (If you are not sure whether or not your shoulders are relaxed, give a big shrug and let your shoulders fall into place).
2. Shake out your arms and sit up comfortably.
3. Place your upper arms close to your side.
4. Bend your elbows so that your upper arm and forearm make a right angle at the elbow.
5. Extend your wrists as described in the previous chapter.

(Examples of sitting and carrying in this position are illustrated on the last page of this chapter.)

Chapter 10: A BETTER POSITION

This is the position that the body likes and the one which puts the least stress on the body. The more that the arms, hand and wrists deviate from this position, the more stressful it is for the body.(Keeping the arms close to your sides is a very good idea whether you are carrying a box or working at your desk.)

NOTE: Watch for those sharp edges where you rest or place your wrists. The wrist bones (carpals) together with the working surface's sharp edge can cause compression of the nerve.

Once you have arrived at the proper position, you will probably find that some of the equipment at your work station isn't easily accessible. Perhaps the equipment is too low, or too high, or the placement of certain objects needs to change. The good news is that there are wonderful and varied devices that are available to help you to work comfortably.

There are many catalogs that carry ergonomic, state-of-the-art equipment. There are a couple of things to consider before you buy: (1) Find items that are

Section III: RELIEF AND PREVENTION

---

adjustable so that you have the greatest range of possibilities for a proper fit; (2) Verify that the company has a liberal return policy. You are unique. Something might sound appropriate for you to use, but if you feel uncomfortable after using it a few days, you'll want to be able to exchange or return the item without a hassle. Just don't give up experimenting. Be patient. There *is* a just-right work station environment to serve you.

Chapter 10: A BETTER POSITION

CORRECT CARRYING POSITION

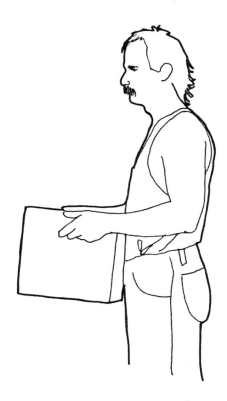

Chapter 10: A BETTER POSITION

CORRECT SITTING POSITION

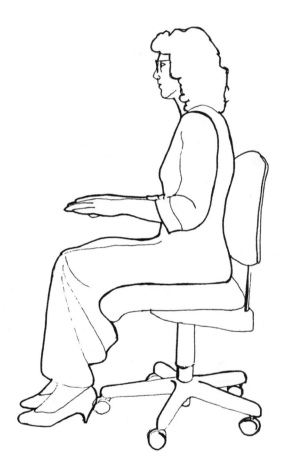

Chapter 11

YOU ARE WHAT YOU EAT

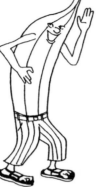

As I stated in a previous chapter, stress is a component of health. So is nutrition. The adage, "You are what you eat," is at work all of the time.

In nutrition, we hear a lot about the "bad stuff." It seems that with all the information about fats and cholesterol, children under three years of age are the only ones who do not know about food culprits. But, what about the "good stuff?" You know, those foods and nutritional supplements that are our friends and allies in life.

There have been studies on nutrition as it relates to carpal tunnel syndrome and some interesting positive results have been noted. The vitamin that has been isolated as being effective in the treatment of carpal tunnel syndrome is B-6 (also known as pyridoxine). It seems to be particularly effective when combined with B-2 (riboflavin).

In Chapter 5, when I described the tendons, I mentioned that the tendons have sheaths (synovial sheaths) to lubricate them. When these sheaths don't

Chapter 11: YOU ARE WHAT YOU EAT

have enough lubrication (synovial fluid), then a pattern of irritation and inflammation occurs. The use of vitamin B-6 plays an important role in the production of synovial fluid. Without getting too technical, it also seems that vitamin B-2 helps with the body's use of vitamin B-6.

Do you need to take a vitamin? That is a personal decision. However, I do want to tell you that even though vitamin B-6 is in most foods, it is negatively affected by long storage, canning, roasting, stewing and food-processing. For example, canned salmon loses more than one-half of Vitamin B-6 and frozen vegetables lose up to 44 percent. Additionally, there is evidence that ingesting alcohol, estrogen, anti-depressants, or oral contraceptives can lead to increased needs for vitamin B-6.

If you do decide to use a supplement, you may want to discuss the type and the potency with your physician.

Remember this about nutrition or nutritional supplements: if you decide to try nutrition, be patient. It can take 90 days or so to really notice results. Good results can begin so subtly that you may not notice right away the diminishing times of discomfort. One client

Sources of Vitamin B-6 (Pyridoxine)

All foods contain some Vitamin B-6. Here are some of the foods considered to be highest in the vitamin:

FRUITS	VEGS.	MEATS	MISC.

Highest group:

	Carrots	Chicken	Wheat germ
	Peas	Beef	Brewer's
	Spinach	Fish	yeast
			Sunflower
			seeds
			Walnuts
			Eggs

Next highest group:

Avocado	Beans		Blackstrap
Bananas	Cabbage		molasses
Cantaloupe			Whole grains

said that he went home one night realizing that something was different about the day, but it wasn't until bedtime that he realized he had been free from pain for the entire time.

Before I close this chapter, I want to remind you of the importance of water. Not fluids, but **water.** When the body does not have enough water to do all that the body needs to do with water, it has to make decisions. The body will make decisions in terms of survival. It will not be nearly as concerned with the manufacture of synovial fluid to lubricate the tendons as it will with something life threatening such as maintaining body temperature by sweating.

Please do not ask the body to choose. Make sure that you are drinking sufficient water everyday.

Chapter 12

EXTENDING YOUR REACH

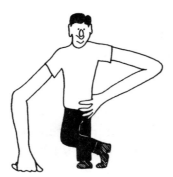

Stretching is one of my favorite subjects. I suspect that I like stretching because it does so many good things for us. For that matter, it helps many of the other creatures with whom we share the earth.

For example, ever noticed how much your dog or cat stretches? Personally, I have a bird. When this guy wakes up from a nap, he stretches one wing and then the other followed by stretching one leg and then the other. I have also noticed that during the day, from time to time, he will stretch.

Ever noticed how much children stretch? They stretch after a nap or for no apparent reason during a day. It feels good and feels necessary.

Why do children and animals feel the need to stretch? Let's look at the monarch of stretching - the cat. Picture a cat stretching his front legs. The front paws are extended, the back is up, and at the height of the stretch the front claws are unsheathed and extended. This is preparation for the skills necessary to pounce.

Chapter 12: EXTENDING YOUR REACH

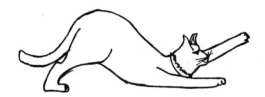

The poor cat would be in a terrible fix if he didn't keep his muscles ready. He might miss the split-second that he needs to reach out, unsheathe his claws and snag a prey.

Stretching gives the cat greater flexibility which, in turn, increases the range of motion in his joints. So, now his joints can move with ease and he has increased the activities available to him. When he stretches, the muscles, tendons, ligaments and joints are being prepared in slow motion for the call to action.

What about you? Do you prepare the muscles, tendons, ligaments and joints for the time when you will want to call them into action? Yes, I know, you stretch every morning for 10 minutes. That's great! That is a step in the right direction. Remember that stretching is done by children and animals **all during the day.**

Muscles do two things: expand or contract. Let's suppose that you have been sitting and working for awhile. Certain muscles have been in a contracted position and others in an expanded position; they need a

Section III: RELIEF AND PREVENTION

break. They also need an opportunity to extend to their full range.

Stretching needs to be done frequently during the day. Perhaps you are thinking that you already have a very busy schedule and do not need more things to do. Well, the nice thing about stretching is that it can be incorporated so easily into a day. Right now, as you are sitting and reading this book, put your arms behind your back . Grab your right wrist with your left hand and lightly pull. Now, repeat with the other arm. Think of all the times and places during a day that you could do that simple stretch.

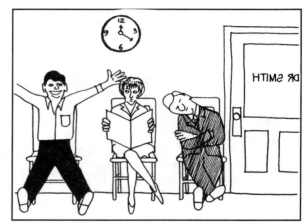

Consider all the mini-vacations from your work station that you have. What are you doing on the trip to refill your water glass? What are you doing while you wait for the copies from the photocopier? What are you doing when you're waiting in line at the postoffice...the market...the traffic signal?

Chapter 12: EXTENDING YOUR REACH

In one of my workshops, I demonstrate a whole stretch routine that includes most of the major muscles of the legs and back and can be done while sitting in a chair. I do not want to leave you with the impression that you need to do a whole routine every time you stretch. You can do different and specific stretches depending upon the position you have held for awhile or the movement you have been doing.

Stretching does have a few rules:

(1) Avoid bouncing while stretching.
(2) Stretch very slowly and deliberately so that you can easily feel the extent of the stretch. (Think of the cat.)
(3) Most stretches only need to be held 10-15 seconds.
(4) If you do not feel stretched out enough, rather than holding the stretch for a long time, let the muscles contract and then stretch again.
(5) If it hurts, *don't* do it.

This little bit of effort can be a wonderful tool for your prevention kit. **Stretching not only increases flexibility but also makes you less prone to injury.**

Section III: RELIEF AND PREVENTION

At the end of this chapter there are some stretches for the fingers, hands, wrists and forearms. There is also an order form for the stretching and strengthening chart at the back of the book. You can post the chart at your work station as a reminder to take care of yourself. After all, with 15 seconds per stretch, you could do six stretches and spend only one and a half minutes. Isn't that a good return on your time investment?

Chapter 12: EXTENDING YOUR REACH

Fingers, Hands and Forearms
Stretches

Before you start a stretching routine, remember the following about stretching:

❑ This is not a contest to see how far and fast you can stretch. Stretch *s-l-o-w-l-y* so that you can feel the limit of the stretch. Come out of the stretch just as slowly as you went into it.

❑ Stretching is more effective if you are warmed up. In the morning, try doing your stretches in the shower or right after you shower.

❑ Cultivate a peaceful state of mind while you are stretching. Once you have a routine, concentrate on your breathing while stretching.

❑ Stretches involving the forearms, hands and fingers do not need to be held for more than 10-15 seconds.

❑ Avoid bouncy or jerky movements when stretching or when holding a stretch.

Section III: RELIEF AND PREVENTION

The Stretches

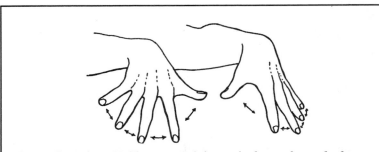

Finger Stretches: Hold arms straight out in front of your body. Bend your wrists down and stretch your fingers out as far as possible. Hold for 12 seconds. Relax and repeat one more time.

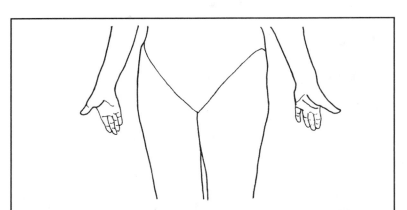

Hand/Forearm Stretch: Place hands at sides with palms down and thumbs facing out. Push palms down to stretch forearms.

Chapter 12: EXTENDING YOUR REACH

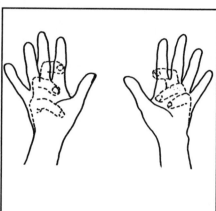

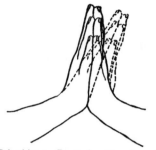

Wrist/Arm Stretch: Bend wrist up to form almost a right angle to arm. With fingers of other hand, slowly push finger of bent hand back towards wrist. Repeat with other hand.

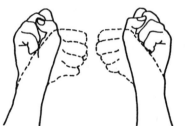

Finger/Wrist Flexing: Curl fingers into palms beginning with little finger. Make a complete fist by rolling thumbs in also. Then curl wrists.

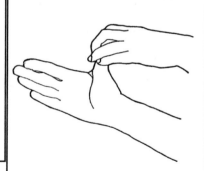

Thumb Stretch: Place hand on side with little finger down and thumb up. Grasp thumb with other hand and pull *GENTLY* away from palm. Repeat with other hand.

Chapter 13

BUILDING UP INSTEAD OF TEARING DOWN

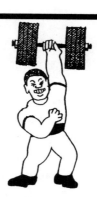

As I mentioned in the previous chapter, when we stretch we lengthen the muscle fiber and increase flexibility. When we exercise, we add muscle fiber and increase strength and stamina.

Strengthening is another factor in avoiding injury. Whereas stretching gives us the flexibility, strengthening keeps us from tiring so quickly. *When we are tired, we tend to make poor judgements which can lead to accidents. We also overwork the muscle which can lead to strains and sprains.*

Stretching   =   Increased Flexibility

Strengthening =   Increased Stamina

As with stretching, strengthening can be done with a minimum commitment of time. In workshops, I often suggest that strengthening movements be done when a mini-vacation for the hands is taking place. Those times might be when we are on hold for a phone connection or when we are watching T.V.

Section III: RELIEF AND PREVENTION

The type of exercise that is most often suggested for the hands, fingers and forearms is the resistance type. Resistance for hands usually means placing some object in the palm and squeezing. This will exercise the hands and forearms. Then the object is placed between the thumbs and individual fingers to exercise the fingers as well as the tendons and muscles that provide movement to the fingers. There are some examples of each at the back of this chapter.There are also some examples of strengthening exercises when you do not have an object available.

 The types of objects that some people like to use (such as grippers and hard putty balls) may be fine for boxers or weight lifters but they are too resistant for most people. For most of us, the hands and arms tire so quickly that we do not really develop the stamina and muscle fiber growth that we are trying to achieve.

It would be better to use an object that you can squeeze many times before the hand or fingers tire. The object , usually a ball, should quickly return to its original form. I provide a foam ball to each of the attendees in the workshop and that seems to work well.

Chapter 13: BUILDING UP...

What really surprises people when they begin to exercise their fingers is the lack of strength in their little finger. For those of you who have used a manual typewriter, perhaps you remember how difficult it was to press down on the keys with your little finger. In those days, if the typing involved carbon duplicates which, in turn, depended upon pressure, you could see the difference in strength from the index finger to the little finger. There would be bold, clear letters where the index finger had punched the keys, but where the little finger had been in charge, the type was almost unreadable. After you worked on the typewriter for awhile, you gained considerable strength in your smallest fingers and you might have strengthened it to the point that you could not tell any difference in pressure on the carbon copies. The same thing happens with the strengthening exercises.

 A word of caution: If you are reading this book because you already have wrist problems, it might be better if you leave out the strengthening exercises until you have done all the other preventive measures and have begun to feel improvement. The reasoning is that if the muscles are already inflamed or irritated, working them harder can aggravate the problem.

Section III: RELIEF AND PREVENTION

For those who are not having a problem and are reading this book solely to prevent problems, there is also a word of caution:

Once your hand, fingers or forearm begin to tire, **stop exercising.** There is plenty of time to develop the muscles. The best way to build the muscle is to spend short and more frequent times at the exercises. Above all, do not follow the "No pain, no gain" approach.

Chapter 13: BUILDING UP ...

Strengthening Exercises
(with a ball)

Developing strength in the arms and hands can help prevent injury. In these exercises, resistance is provided by a foam rubber ball.

Place the ball in the palm of your hand and squeeze using all fingers and thumb. Continue to squeeze and release until your hand tires. Repeat with other hand.

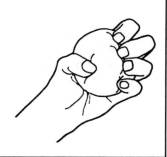

Pinch the ball between your index finger and thumb 10 times. Then pinch the ball between your middle finger and thumb 10 times. Continue until each finger has been exercised. Repeat with other hand.

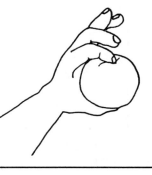

 If you experience pain or discomfort doing these exercises, STOP IMMEDIATELY

Section III: RELIEF AND PREVENTION

STRENGTHENING EXERCISES
(without a ball)

These exercises provide elements of stretching, flexing and range of motion. They can be done anywhere and don't require any devices to help you.

IF YOU EXPERIENCE PAIN OR DISCOMFORT WHILE DOING THESE EXERCISES, **STOP IMMEDIATELY!**

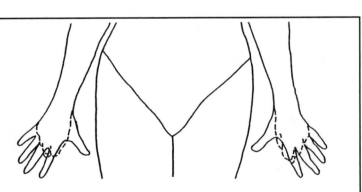

Place arms at your sides with thumbs pointing towards your body. Stretch fingers as far apart as possible. Then make a fist and hold for 12 seconds. Relax and repeat.

STRENGTHENING EXERCISES (CONTINUED)
(without a ball)

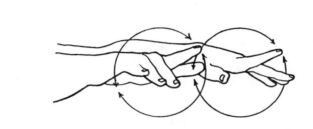

Hold arms straight in front of your body. Keeping wrists straight, draw circles with your index fingers rotating your wrists at the same time. Circle in each direction 5 times.

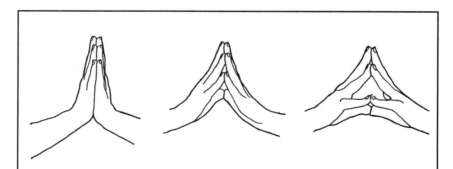

Place hands in prayer position. Extend thumbs. Open fingers slowly while pushing on fingertips. Spread fingers as far as they will comfortably go.

Chapter 14

KNEADING A RUB

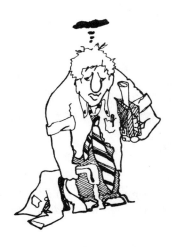

Remember in an earlier chapter, I mentioned that while I was learning massage my arms and fingers would ache? Besides changing my wrist posture and movements, I also went to other students and asked them to work on my arms and hands. There was one fellow who had very strong hands. He could really bear down on my arms. The next day, I would feel a little sore, but the relief was dramatic. I wholly recommend massage to you.

The role of massage in prevention is important. Not only can massage often relieve pain, but it can also stimulate circulation, prevent edema and help maintain your mobility. If you find a massage therapist who understands the mechanics of carpal tunnel syndrome well, he or she can easily spend an hour working from the fingers up the arm to the shoulder and the neck. As I stated earlier in the book, the place where you are feeling discomfort may not be the source and a knowledgeable massage therapist will want to consider all of the pathways.

Chapter 14: KNEADING A RUB

Perhaps the idea of someone you don't know touching you is not OK. Perhaps you cannot afford massage sessions. No problem. There are some things that you can do for yourself. They may not be as effective as a professional can do, but there is still a lot you can do. One of the positive aspects of the hands and forearms, unlike the back, is that you can reach all of the places.

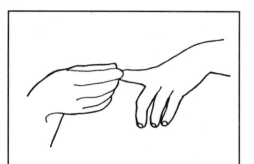

One of the positive aspects of the hands and forearms...is that you can reach all of the places.

Sometimes people feel uneasy about self-massage. They are not sure what they should do. At the end of the chapter, I have given a suggested massage routine for you to do on yourself (or to have someone do for you). You will notice that your arms, hands and fingers will tingle and come to life after you complete the massage.

Don't hold back. Approach your arms, hands and fingers with confidence. After all, think about what little workhorses those hands and fingers are every day. They can take, and they like, a lot of pressure. You

Section III: RELIEF AND PREVENTION

might have to go a little lighter on the forearms though, especially if there is pain.

I can honestly tell you that your hands and fingers will feel refreshed if you take a mini-vacation and massage them. Doing a mini-massage on your hands and fingers has the additional bonus of enlivening your whole self.

Benefits of Massage

❑ Reduction in inflammation

❑ Increase in range of motion

❑ Heightened blood circulation

❑ Lessening of mental stress

❑ Release of muscle tension

❑ Improved body metabolism

❑ Renewal of energy

❑ Heightened physical awareness

❑ It feels good!

Section III: RELIEF AND PREVENTION

Fingers, Hands and Forearms
Massage

Massage can provide relief from pain, stimulate circulation, prevent edema and maintain mobility. Here is a routine that you can do for yourself:

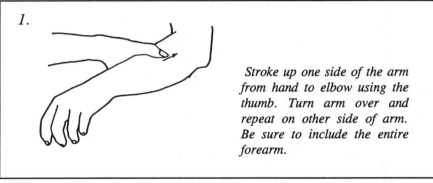

1.

Stroke up one side of the arm from hand to elbow using the thumb. Turn arm over and repeat on other side of arm. Be sure to include the entire forearm.

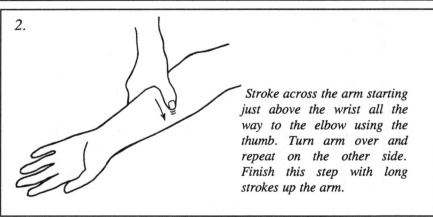

2.

Stroke across the arm starting just above the wrist all the way to the elbow using the thumb. Turn arm over and repeat on the other side. Finish this step with long strokes up the arm.

Chapter 14: KNEADING A RUB

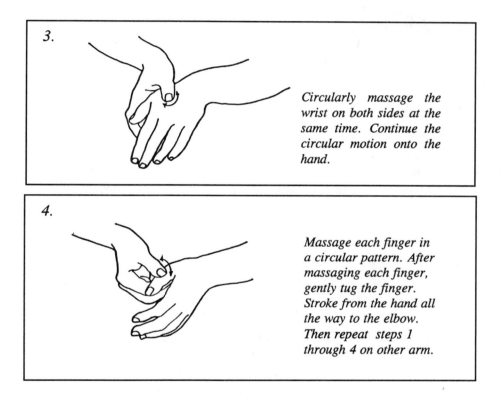

3. Circularly massage the wrist on both sides at the same time. Continue the circular motion onto the hand.

4. Massage each finger in a circular pattern. After massaging each finger, gently tug the finger. Stroke from the hand all the way to the elbow. Then repeat steps 1 through 4 on other arm.

Use this routine, alter it, or make up one of your own. In any case, your forearms, hands and fingers will feel refreshed and will thank you for the mini-vacation.

Chapter 15

MY HAND'S ON THE TRIGGER

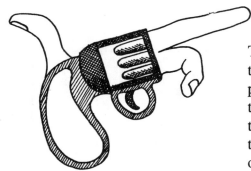

There is a form of effective therapy called "trigger point" therapy. The reason that it has the name of trigger point is because it is the place where pain shoots out to other places.

A few times in this book, I have said that sometimes the place where we feel discomfort or pain is not the source. What is happening is that the pain is "referring" from a point - the trigger point.

Trigger points are places in a muscle that are hyperirritable spots and they trigger the pain to other places.

There has been quite a bit of medical mapping of these points. The best known work on the subject was done by Dr. Travell and Dr. Simons. There are even wall charts showing the areas of referred pain and the associated trigger point. Since this book is about taking care of yourself, I would like to give you some ideas on how you can use trigger point therapy without needing to learn all about the medical mapping.

Chapter 15: MY HAND'S ON THE TRIGGER

Before a discussion of the way to do trigger point therapy on yourself, I would like to go over some of the times when trigger point work would be especially useful. Those times are:

(1) When your pain increases as you do stretches.
(2) When muscles are weak and exercise doesn't seem to be strengthening them.
(3) When you are experiencing decreased range of movement.
(4) When you have tenderness at the trigger point.
(5) When you have referred pain.
(6) When the muscle is under stress.

 (If you have any of the above conditions and trigger point work does not help, you may want to check with the appropriate physician.)

Here again, as with massage, the nice thing is that you can reach all of the areas of your forearms. My personal preference is to do this therapy after the massage. That way, I can more easily identify the trigger point spots. In time, as you become more sensitive to the feel of your muscles, you may notice a small knot in a muscle. This is often the trigger point.

Section III: RELIEF AND PREVENTION

The way to begin is to use the thumb or finger of the other hand, and press down along the fingers, hands and arms locating really painful spots. When you find a very irritated point, push in on it. To determine how deep to push, let me give you the method that I use in my practice:

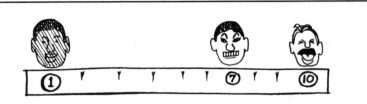

I use the zero to 10 rating system. No pain is zero and 10 is the opposite extreme. Apply pressure on the spot in the 7 to 8 range.

Keep your pressure steady as you continue to push on the spot for 30 seconds to one minute (depending on how soon the pain disappears and the muscle relaxes.) While you are holding the spot, breath deeply and steadily. With every inhalation, visualize sending oxygen to the place where you are applying pressure. Remember to keep your pressure steady.

Chapter 15: MY HAND'S ON THE TRIGGER

During that time, if you are on the correct spot, you will feel the pain diminish and even go away. If there is no change or if the pain worsens, then you have found a referred area and not the trigger point.

Sometimes when I apply this technique and I am right on the trigger point, the relief will occur immediately. Go ahead and try it.

Section III: RELIEF AND PREVENTION

Trigger Point Therapy

Trigger point therapy is very effective. It can be useful in many circumstances, such as:

1. When the pain is dull and aching.
2. When the pain is deep.
3. When pressure on the trigger point causes pain or increases pain.
4. When the muscles are tight or cramped.

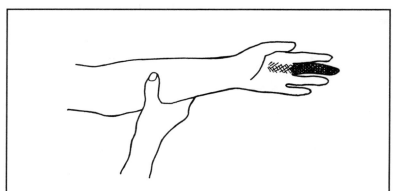

Rarely is the pain located at the same place as the trigger point. In the above illustration, the painful area is indicated by the shaded area, yet the source is up on the forearm.

Chapter 15: MY HAND'S ON THE TRIGGER

Here are some more illustrations showing examples of the trigger points (indicated by "o") and the areas of referred pain (indicated by shading):

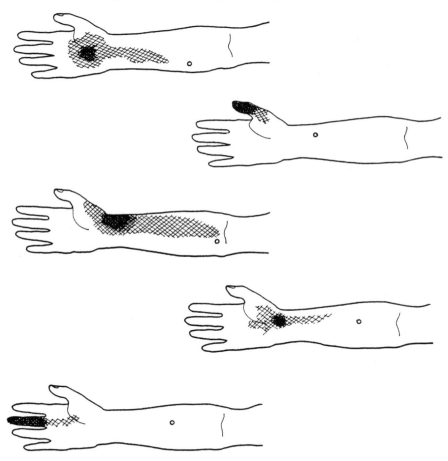

SECTION IV

PLANNING

and

MOTIVATION

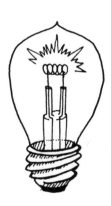

Chapter 16

THE ROADMAP

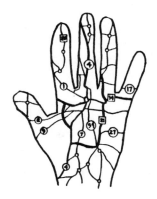

It is difficult to do all of the prevention techniques at the same time. It would be difficult to remember even three at a time. Let me give you some suggestions as to an order.

Two prevention techniques that can be done right away and can make a great deal of difference are correcting your posture and the way you hold your wrists. After this analysis, you will be in a good position to realize what changes you need to make in your environment and equipment to support you correctly.

The next possible step would be to begin to change your nutrition or to take the nutritional supplements. The earlier you begin, the better. It sometimes takes awhile to notice any significant changes.

Little by little, you can start learning. Try adding stretching and strengthening exercises to your daily routine. Find those little bits of time to use for creating new health habits. At the end of this chapter is a form you can photocopy and complete to create a program for your self. One of the best ways to remember is to paste a sticky note in an obvious place. At the end of this book is a form you can also complete to obtain a stretching and strengthening chart to put up on the wall at home or in your office to help you remember to take care of yourself.

There are always stressors to resolve. This is a big task, but you can do it. Start by paying attention to your body's needs. When your arms and hands are tired, give yourself a mini-massage and then check for trigger points. Resolve to treat yourself kindly.

These are some suggestions for you. You can use the plan at the back of this chapter or create one of you own. The important part is that you have a plan to keep yourself well. Life goes so much better when you feel good.

Here's an example of a chart that you can prepare to help you. Once you have planned the time of day and the activity that you can do at that time, mark an "x" in the box where the time and activity meet. The extra box at each activity is for comments to yourself. Make up a sticky note or paper and tape it to a place to help you remember… the car dash, your computer screen, your locker.

BEST TIMES TO TAKE CARE OF MYSELF

ACTIVITY and COMMENT	In the morning	On the morning commute	During the day	On my breaks	At lunchtime	On the evening commute	At home	At hobbies or sports
Stress								
Mini-vacations								
Ergonomics								
Stretching								
Strengthening								
Massage								
Trigger Points								
Nutrition								
Splinting								
Resting								
Daily Activity								
Other								

Chapter 17
LIGHT AT THE END OF THE CARPAL TUNNEL

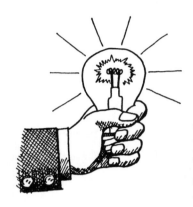

The saddest stories of carpal tunnel sydrome that I hear involve the person who procrastinated until all the doctor can recommend is surgery coupled with a change in lifestyle and job. By that time, the person is concerned enough to take action because he or she wants relief from the pain. Usually the story goes that there was a little discomfort now and then - nothing serious and it was possible to override the discomfort. That isn't much of a victory and it is usually short lived. The pain may retreat for awhile but it will be back and perhaps be worse.

 Try not to let the situation get beyond your control. As you have learned in this book, there are many things that you can do to help yourself.

On the next page, let's look at the areas that can be changed and that can help your body do better.

Chapter 17: LIGHT AT THE END...

THE THINGS THAT I CAN DO TO HELP MYSELF
ARE:

❑ Noting where my body is feeling discomfort or
pain.

❑ Varying my tasks more and taking breaks from
my work station.

❑ Recognizing and taking action to eliminate
stressors.

❑ Protecting my wrist posture while I am sleeping.

❑ Observing any wrist deviations, the degree and
frequency.

❑ Correcting my use of work station/tools as
required.

❑ Obtaining the necessary ergonomic devices to
help me at my work station.

❑ Paying attention to my overall shoulder and arm
posture.

❑ Taking in the necessary nutrients and water.

Section IV: PLANNING AND MOTIVATION

- ❑   Stretching my body throughout the day.

- ❑   Strengthening my body through resistance exercise.

- ❑   Stimulating my muscles through massage.

- ❑   Using trigger point therapy to provide relief.

Start now. Begin with observation and work your way through the previous list of suggestions to provide a complete prevention program for yourself. You have everything to gain in keeping and maintaining your health for as long as you live.

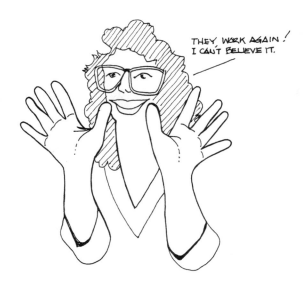

GLOSSARY

acute: having a short and rather severe course

carpals: the bones of the wrist

carpal tunnel: wrist tunnel which is the passageway for the median nerve and the tendons that flex your fingers

cartilage: specialzed, fibrous connective tissue

chronic: long duration or frequent recurrence

compression: squeezing together; action exerted upon a body which tends to increase its density

congenital: existing at birth

contract (muscle): to draw shorter and broader

cumulative trauma disorders: type of injury usually developing gradually as a result of repeated microtrauma

deviation: a turning away or aside from the normal point

diagnosis: identifying a disease by its signs or symptoms

english: releasing a motion to produce a rotary or spin to an object

expand: to increase in size

flexibility: readily bent without breaking

flexor tenosynovitis: inflammation of the tendons and enveloping sheath of the muscles whose action is to flex a joint

health: the condition of being sound in body, mind and soul; freedom from physical disease or pain.

GLOSSARY

hypochondriac: someone who believes in their imaginary physical illnesses

inflammation: a local response to an injury of swelling, redness, pain, and heat

ligament: a tough band of tissue connecting bone to bone

massage: systematic therapeutic friction, stroking and kneading of the body

mobility: capacity to move or be moved

median nerve: nerve that exits the spinal column at the neck and continues down the shoulder, upper arm and carpal tunnel to the thumb, middle, index fingers and part of the ring finger

muscles: tissues that are capable of contracting and function to produce motion

muscle fiber: the tissue that contracts when stimulated

nerves: tissue that when stimulated carries impulses to act

nutrition: the process by which food is taken in and processed

nutritional supplements: something that completes or makes an addition to food

pinched nerve: a nerve which is being squeezed or compressed painfully

predisposing conditions: to be susceptible or inclined to a certain disease or disorder

prevention: to take act in advance against something happening

GLOSSARY

---

pronator teres syndrome: a condition in which the median nerve is compressed by the heads of the pronator teres muscle

referred pain: pain felt in a part of the body at some distance from its cause

regenerate: to form or create again

relief: removal or lessening of pain or distress

repetitive motion injury: the pain or discomfort experienced when repeated movement thickens the tendons' lubricating membranes thereby squeezing nerves against bone and ligament

resistance (muscle): to exert force in opposition to the muscle

rigidity: lacking flexibility; stiff, hard

signs: objective evidence of disease

spasms: involuntary and abnormal muscle contraction

splint: material or device used to protect/immobilize a body part

stamina: staying power, endurance

steroids: a group name for a large family of lipids which include, in part, progesterone, gonadal hormones and adrenocortical hormones

strength (training): power to resist force

stress: bodily or mental tension that maybe a factor in disease

stretching: extending the body or limbs

GLOSSARY

surgery: branch of medicine which treats diseases, injuries and deformities by operation or manipulation

symptoms: subjective evidence of disease

syndromes: a group of signs and symptoms that occur together and are characteristic of a certain disease or disorder

synovial sheath: the membrane containing the lubricating fluid secreted for the tendons

systemic: affecting the whole body

tendons: the band or cord that unites a muscle to bone and transmits the force which the muscle exerts

thoracic outlet syndrome: a condition in which poor neck and shoulder posture or a cervical rib put pressure on the nerve root which passes from the neck to the arm

trigger points: a small place on a muscle which turns on a relatively larger output of pain or discomfort

twinges: a sudden, sharp local pain

variety: changing from time to time

vitamin: organic substances that are essential to the body in small quantities and act in the regulation of metabolic processes

vitamin B-2 (riboflavin): heat-stable factor of Vitamin B complex; acts as component of two coenzymes which function as hydrogen carriers in oxidation-reduction processes; found in milk, muscle, liver, kidney, eggs, grass, malt, leafy young vegetables and various algae

GLOSSARY

---

vitamin B-6 (pyridoxine): associated with the utilization of unsaturated fatty acids; in humans, deficiency may result in increased irritability, convulsions and peripheral neuritis; found in brewer's yeast, wheat bran, wheat germ, milk, cantaloupe, liver, kidney, heart, cabbage, eggs, beef and black - strap molasses.

water: the liquid that is a major part of all living matter

INDEX

INDEX

Flexor tenosynovitis, 47
Forearms, 17, 24, 39-40, 64, 72, 86, 92, 94, 99-100

G-H

Gout, 21
Hands, 17, 24, 39-41, 45-47, 52, 58, 65, 67, 73, 84, 86, 92, 94, 99-100, 106, 114
Health, 78, 113, 118
Hobbies, 27, 50
Hypothyroidism, 21

I-J

Immobilization, 53
Injury, 26-27, 28, 85, 91
Joints, 21, 37, 53, 64-66, 83

L

Lifestyle, 54
Ligaments, 41-42, 83

M

Massage, 68, 98-103, 105, 114, 118
  benefits, 101
  routine, 102-103
Medicine:
  drugs, 53-54
  profession, 31
Mini-vacations, 21, 24, 27, 84, 100
Movement, 20, 23, 30, 40, 53, 64-68, 72, 92, 98
Movement, range of, 17, 38, 64-65, 83,105
Muscle:
  action, 38-40, 53, 64-65, 83, 92
  fatigue, 20, 25-27, 32
  fiber, 91-92
  hyperirritable, 104
  inflammation, 26, 31, 46, 66-67, 93
  regeneration, 25-26, 94
  spasms, 29,
  weak, 105

INDEX

N

Neck, 41, 45-46, 98
Nerves, 21, 26, 41, 45-46, 52
  median (middle nerve), 41,
Numbness in hands, 17, 44, 47, 58
Nutrition, 78-80, 117
 supplements, 78-79

O-P

Osteopaths, 51
Overuse, 26
Pain, 52, 60, 116-117
  acute, 30
  chronic, 30-31
  referred, 46, 104-109
Palms, 40, 52, 69, 92
Planning (routine), 113-115
Positions, 64, 67, 70-71, 72-73
  carrying, 72-73, 75
  neutral, 64-65
  sitting, 72-73, 77

Posture, 20, 32, 72, 98, 113, 117
Predisposing conditions, 18, 20-21, 30
Pregnancy, 20
Professional help, 49-51
Pronator teres syndrome, 47

R

Repetitve motion injuries, 32, 50,
Repetition, 21-22, 24-25, 32, 66-67
Rest, 21, 24, 27, 32, 61
Resistance, 92
Rheumatoid arthritis, 21
Room temperatures, 21

S

Shoulder, 41, 45-46, 72, 98
Signs, 44
Sleep, 29, 59, 68, 117
Splints, 53-54, 69

INDEX

BIOGRAPHICAL SKETCH

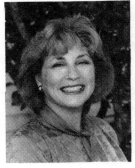

Rosemarie Atencio is a health practitioner, writer, workshop leader and consultant. She contracts with companies, organizations and associations to provide wellness workshops, ergonomic consulting, and health programs.

Rosemarie received her training in San Diego, California. After completing her internship at a medical clinic, she graduated as a holistic health practitioner. Her training included anatomy, physiology, kinesiology, psychology, stress management, massage, exercise, nutrition, health and ergonomics.

From consulting in her private practice, she developed wellness workshops for businesses. She realized that if you can educate someone on the "how-to" of taking care of themselves, then injuries and accidents could be reduced. It was out of the experiences of one of these workshops entitled "It's All in the Wrists" that Rosemarie wrote this book.

Gifts to Give to Yourself and Others...

The Book:
CARPAL TUNNEL SYNDROME: How to Relieve and Prevent Wrist "Burnout" by Rosemarie Atencio.
Designed with you in mind. Whatever your occupation, profession or job, this book is crammed with good ideas for the care of your hands, wrist and forearms.
$13.95 plus shipping & handling *

The Video Tape:
CARPAL TUNNEL SYNDROME: How to Relieve and Prevent Wrist "Burnout" by Rosemarie Atencio and Stan Hall.
Practical, easy-to-follow demonstrations of stretching, strengthening, massage, and correct wrist movements .
$21.95 plus shipping & handling*

The Poster:
Stretching and Strengthening to Prevent Wrist "Burnout" by Rosemarie Atencio.
Laminated 8 1/2 x 11 poster for office, home or anywhere else you need to have a reminder.
$4.95 plus shipping & handling * (Black & White)
$11.95 plus shipping & handling (Color)

---

*Special Offer: Buy the Book and the Video at the same time and get a black and white laminated poster FREE!....a SAVINGS OF $4.95!

The Newsletter: *
NoStress Newsletter by Health & Wellness Dynamics
Quick and easy to read newsletter with articles on stress, nutrition, exercise, and ergonomics.
$3.85 for a 1-year subscription (6 issues) Rate includes postage. Call for quantity rates.

   After you've read the book , give us your opinion and we'll send you a FREE 1 year's subscription to the *NoStress Newsletter.*
*(*see next page for details)

Fill out this portion to order orto receive your FREE Subscription

Company:_____

Your name:_____

Title:_____

Address: _____

City:_____ State_____ Zip_____

Phone:_____Fax_____

I found the book to be: _____

_____

_____

May we quote you? ☐ Yes   ☐ No

Order Form

Item	Price	Quantity	Total
The Book: Carpal Tunnel Syndrome	$13.95		
The Tape: Carpal Tunnel Syndrome	$21.95		
Tape and Book AND FREE B/W Laminated Poster	$35.90		
The Poster: Stretching and Strengthening (B/W)	$ 4.95		
Stretching and Strengthening (color)	11.95		

For VISA/Mastercard, call 1+800-935-7323 .
Send check or money order (do not send cash) to:

HWD Publishing, PO Box 220, Veneta, OR 97487.

(Call for quantity discounts) (503) 935-1608

Subtotal: $ _____

Shipping/Handling: $3.50 _____

Total: $ _____

Allow 2-3 weeks for delivery

Satisfaction guaranteed or your money will be refunded.